BRETT MARTY

MUSCLES

The Ultimate Guide on How to Build Muscle Mass, Learn the Secrets for the Right Diet and Effective Workout Techniques That Would Guarantee Muscle Gain

Descrierea CIP a Bibliotecii Naționale a României
BRETT MARTY
   MUSCLES. The Ultimate Guide on How to Build Muscle Mass, Learn the Secrets for the Right Diet and Effective Workout Techniques That Would Guarantee Muscle Gain / Brett Marty – Bucharest: Editura My Ebook, 2021
   ISBN

BRETT MARTY

MUSCLES

The Ultimate Guide on How to Build Muscle Mass, Learn the Secrets for the Right Diet and Effective Workout Techniques That Would Guarantee Muscle Gain

My Ebook Publishing House
Bucharest, 2021

TABLE OF CONTENTS

MIND-SET CONDITIONING

Stop Giving Excuses

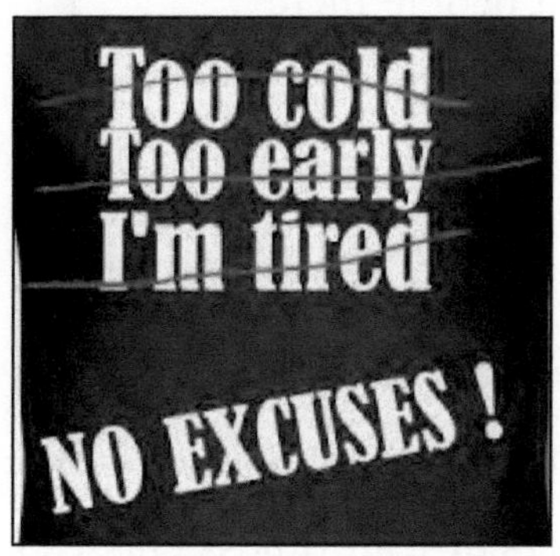

"You can have results or excuses. Not both."

Road blocks, brick walls, obstacles, bumps in the road, reasons or whatever you call them - they exist and they get in our way daily in our quest to be healthy and fit.

Stop giving excuses. Never let them hinder your quest for the healthier and happier life. Also, due to the present access to high calorific food, the fitness excuses that one ensured our survival, now send us to an early grave. The best way to get back on board is to stop making excuses.

Below I've provided the 5 most common fitness excuses people use to avoid exercising:

- I don't have enough time

- I have no motivation to workout

- I feel intimidated by the fit people there

- I don't have anyone to train with

- The gym is too expensive or far

These are some of the standard excuses for not making it to the gym that can be heard around the office, school or park every day. Those who are personal trainers or lead fitness classes know the excuses can be much more creative.

To achieve your health and fitness goals, you have to stop making excuses. Not just that, your mindset plays a significant role as well. A positive mindset is the most powerful tool for reaching your goals. The way you perceive your fitness journey will either make or break your goals.

The Power Of Mindset

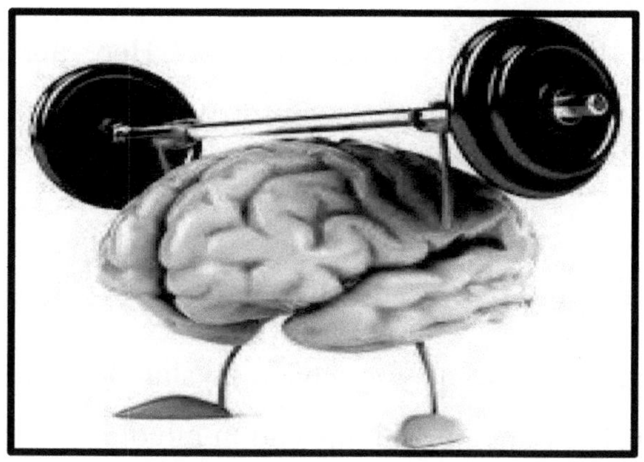

Fitness begins with the mind, not the body. Never underestimate the power of your mind. The mind has always been at the core of building muscle. Hence, before adhering to any fitness program, the first Muscle Gain Secrets is to get your mindset right. Clear all negative thinking and replace them with positive ones to empower your muscle building journey. Understand that your thoughts are what hold you back from what you truly want to achieve.

The essentiality of having a strong mind is often overshadowed by being strong physically. If you have the right mindset, you will have the mental power to stay focused and push yourself, even when things get tough. Not having the right mindset will result in you end up sabotaging your health and fitness goals in many ways.

So how do you 'Fix' your mindset? Here are *5 Simple Techniques* to help you achieve your dream body with the right mindset:

1. Set Goals That Are Both Specific & Achievable

You can only WIN if you have a crystal clear outcome. So remember to always begin with the end in mind.

Ask yourself questions like: What's my ideal weight? How much muscle mass do I want to gain? Is it 10 pounds? 20 pounds? Is my goal only attainable in three months or more? What does it take to achieve my goals? The 2 Rules is to be both Specific & Achievable - do not just estimate or simply see-how-it-goes. It plays an important part in holding yourself accountable to the goals you set.

Without setting specific and achievable goals, you are more likely to stumble and fail. Make your goals specific, write them down! Then put your list of goals onto your mirror, your fridge, your work table, or even your phone screen - just anything that's clearly visible to you every day. This will keep you reminded of your most important goals every day whether you feel like it or not. In the long-term, this will condition your mind in an empowering way! Mindset conditioning has immense power in fuelling your determination and commitment in your goal to ultimate successful muscle gain.

2. Cultivate Patience

You need time to achieve your desired goals and this requires patience. Be patient for results because muscle gain is not going to happen overnight. Take a step back and evaluate what you have achieved so far. Cultivate patience and learn to celebrate little victories along the way in your goal setting process. This will encourage and motivate you to keep you going.

Everybody is wired differently.

The general rule of thumb is to build 1 pound of muscle per week. Some are able to build more, some less, depending on their diet and exercise regime. So in a month, an average person can expect to put on 1-3 pounds of muscle mass. This gives you a good idea how to set achievable and realistic Goals. If you're expecting to gain 10 pounds in a month, most probably you're putting on more fat than muscle mass.

So many people expect results in a minimal timeframe and then lose interest when their desired body is nowhere to be seen. Nothing comes easily. Eat smart, work hard, and most importantly have the patience for results. Remember that Rome wasn't built in a Day, and so does your body. If you're working with the right muscle gain plan, eventually the results will prove to you all its worth.

3. Hard Work Is Your Only "Shortcut"

There really isn't any shortcut to muscle gaining. Most of the magic bullets you see in the Fitness Industry today are nothing more than marketing gimmicks. The only way to gain muscle is to invest hard work into building and maintaining it. It is always a gradual process so start small and build from there. There is no substitute for hard work in fitness. The only thing you need to get started is the right knowledge, diet plan, and workout regime. From there, all you need is relentless hard work, patience, and determination to stay on track.

So stop looking for quick fixes as most likely you'd end up burning a hole in your pocket and get nothing in return.

4. Everyone Is Different. Don't Compare

Do not compare yourself to others. Everyone is different - the way your body absorbs nutrient and reacts towards workouts you do are different from other people.

Do not look at others' results and think "Why is he/she achieving results faster and better than I do? I worked as hard or even harder but my results are not visible".

Unnecessary comparison brings disappointment and zero help towards your goal. Focus on your own body. Aim for incremental progress until you finally attain your dream body. Remember, nobody else has your body - you do! Focus only on yourself!

5. Be Completely Committed

Muscle Gain is all about Discipline. The ability to consistently take action regardless of how you feel at any moment. To get started on your fitness journey, all you really need to do is to commit once and do it every single day.

Commit yourself 100% for 90 Days (if not more), set short-term achievable goals – the amount of muscle mass you wish to build, and it shall keep you on track working towards the goals.

This mindset helps you to be realistic. You won't expect immediate results but instead, you'll be focusing on the process and duration. Because you understand and is aware that muscle-gaining takes time and effort. When you are mentally prepared to commit to a timeframe, you will persevere through the process.

Here are some strategies to keep you on track when the journey gets too bumpy:

Journaling - It helps you to track of your own progress

Progress Pictures - Super satisfying as you watch your body evolve each day!

Gym / Diet Buddy - Mental and physical support play a big role in helping you stay motivated

MUSCLE GAIN SECRETS 2

MUSCLE PUMPING DIET

High-protein diets such as Zone, Atkins and Sugar Busters were once popular diet plans in the past few decades. While high-protein diet does lead to weight loss, they have an alarming flaw, which leads to unbalanced meal plans that deprive one of other essential nutrients for a healthy body. However, that doesn't have to be the case.

High protein diets are generally suitable for individuals looking to burn fat and lose weight with a caloric deficit. So if you're looking to gain muscles, it's better for you to go for high carbs, with low/moderate protein. Carbohydrates supply you with energy to blast those weights in the gym and also fill in the caloric surplus you need to actually gain weight and build muscles. Furthermore, studies show that high carb, low protein diet can still help you gain an enviable amount of muscle mass.

What Is Protein?

Protein is one of the 3 main macronutrients along with carbohydrate and fat. Protein is the most important source for muscle gaining as it acts as building blocks for muscle fibers. Simply said, without protein, your muscle won't be able to grow. The best sources of protein are lean meat, eggs, cottage cheese, beans, quinoa and many others. We called these foods 'Protein-rich Powerfood' as they are packed with a higher percentage of protein compared to other nutrients.

To have a better understanding of what protein really is, it is a large molecule composed of smaller units known as the amino acids. Today, we can identify 20 types of amino acids. Different types of proteins are actually derived from different combinations of amino acids. This essential macronutrient can be found in any part of the human body. Your organs, hair, skin, nails, eyes, nose, lips are all made up of protein.

Ultimately, there will be no muscle gain without protein.

What Foods Contain Higher Amount Of Protein?

Working out involves breaking down muscle fibers in order to grow bigger and stronger muscles, and protein is required to repair and grow muscle tissues. Also, it's good to note that protein is the final source of energy after both carbohydrates and fats are depleted, making it perfect for those who wish to burn fats and lose weight.

Now that we understood the importance of protein to muscle gain, we shall move on to the food that contains a higher amount of protein, also known as "Protein-rich Powerfood".

Protein is available from both animal and plant sources. The typical

U.S. diet is a mixture of protein sources. Variety in choices will provide an adequate diet. The following are some examples of protein content in some typical foods.

- 3oz. of chicken contains 20g of protein

- 3 oz. of ground beef contains 21g of protein

- 2 oz. of pork chop contains 15g of protein

- ¾ cup of beans contain 11g of protein

- 2 tablespoons of peanut butter contain 8g of protein

- ½ cup of soybeans contain 10g of protein

What About Protein Powders?

Speak to any fitness enthusiasts in the gym, you'll find that most of them consume protein powders as their staple supplements. So what exactly are they? It's actually a popular protein source to help people improve athletic performance and build muscle mass. This is a go-to solution for those who are looking for a quick and convenient source to fill in their daily protein intake requirements to build muscles. Generally, one scoop of protein powder contains about 25g of protein, and 2 scoops can easily make up with one chicken breast. Plus, it's easier to chuck down a bottle of protein shake than digesting one whole chicken breast.

That said, protein powder is an excellent way to supplement your daily protein needs, especially if you're looking to build muscles. Here are the types of proteins you can find in the market today:

1) **Whey Protein Concentrate** – The most common and affordable form of whey protein. Most of them contain lactose. So for those who are lactose-intolerant, stay away from this.

2) **Whey Protein Isolate** – A more concentrated form of whey protein with little to no fat or lactose. This is the number one choice for those with lactose-intolerant and also the purest form of whey protein you can find today. Whey Protein Isolate usually contains zero carbohydrates and zero fats.

3) **Hemp Protein** – A plant-based protein. Perfect for vegans with additional anti-inflammation benefits from included Omega-3 fatty acids with extra fiber for weight loss and gut health.

4) **Pea Protein Powder** – Another plant-based protein. Vegans' favourite.

5) **Soy Protein Powder** – Just like whey protein, you can find them in concentrate and isolate form. This type of protein comes with a different taste and texture for consumers.

Ways To Add More Protein In Everyday Diet

Besides protein powder, you should also learn how to get your protein intake from other sources, including whole food. Here's a list of food that you can consider adding into your everyday diet to hit your daily protein target:

Cheese. Preferably cheese with low fat and high protein such as string cheese. You can have them as snacks on the go or add them to your meals. Some even prefer to melt them on slices of bread and noodles or even grate and add them to mashed potatoes and their favourite meat for variety.

Cottage cheese or ricotta cheese. Another excellent source of casein protein, a slow-digesting protein that drip-feed your muscles for the entire day. You can consume them as is or even add them to your favourite fruits or vegetables for extra sweetness. Preferably go for low-fat cottage cheese.

Milk or soy milk. Milk is considered to be an easy source of protein. However, most milk contain high carbohydrates and fats so you have to pay close attention to the labels.

Yogurt. This is a bodybuilders' choice of dessert. You can add yogurt to your favourite fruits, cereals, and high-protein snacks to create a wholesome, guilt-free snack.

Eggs. You can find some of the purest forms of protein from eggs. Top Bodybuilders over the decades swear by the benefits of consuming eggs daily. Also, eggs are the cheapest source of protein you can get out there and can be cooked in numerous ways. They can be hard-boiled, soft-boiled, scrambled, poached, pan-fried, baked, basted and sunny-side up. Really now, you can never go wrong with eggs.

Nuts, seeds, wheat germ, and oats. These are the secret snacks you can consume for satiety and excellent protein and fat source. These power-food contain so many benefits on top of being an excellent protein source.

Meat and fish. These are the biggest protein sources you can find to pack on some lean, mean muscles mass. However, if you're a vegan, consider other protein sources above such as nuts, quinoa, cheese and many others.

Planning Your Muscle Gain Phase

Athletes who are attempting to add muscle and strength over time don't have the same macronutrient needs as dieters. They will be in a caloric surplus or at a maintenance and most likely have a higher body fat percentage compared to dieters who practice high protein diet.

As mentioned before, research shows that high protein intake doesn't necessarily guarantee muscle gain. In fact, it is shown that the anabolic effect of high protein diets doesn't extend past around 0.8 g/lb. Thus, it is recommended to consume 0.8-1.0 g/lb of protein on a daily basis to reap all the benefits of a high protein diet.

The rest of your diet should be filled with carbohydrates and fats to fill in the caloric gaps. Usually, you consume 400-500 kcal more than your maintenance during muscle gain phase.

So why do you need less protein during muscle gain phase? The simple reason is because more protein is being utilized for energy when you're restricting calories and have a leaner physique. During muscle gain phase, you usually don't meet such conditions. Therefore, you simply don't need as much protein and you'll reap more benefits from eating more carbohydrates and fat.

When planning your daily diet plan, first decide the number of calories needed for your muscle gain phase. After that, decide how much protein you need (0.8-1.0 g/lb), then set aside 20-30% of your calories comes from fat and the rest from carbohydrates.

With a higher amount of carbohydrates and fats allowed into your diet, you can have more energy to carry out strenuous strength training to gain strength and build muscle mass.

Here's a simplified Table to show how you can easily plan out your daily calories intake during both cutting and muscle gain phase.

RECOMMENDED MACRONUTRIENTS	PROTEIN	FAT	CARBOHYDRATE
CUTTING	1.1 – 1.3 grams per pound (2.3 – 2.8 g/ kg) of bodyweight	15 – 25% of total calories per day	The remaining calories are filled with carbs
MUSCLE GAIN	0.8 – 1.0 grams per pound (1.8 – 2.3 g/ kg) of bodyweight	20 – 30% of total calories per da	The remaining calories are filled with carbs

MUSCLE GAIN SECRETS 3

MUST HAVE MUSCLE GAINING SUPPLEMENTS

Significance of Muscle Gaining Supplements

Generally, to build up muscle it is still better to achieve it via diet and exercise while supplementation should only be used for additive effects. Nonetheless, it should not be pushed aside as supplements are still generally used for health and building muscle. The Top 3 most used supplements are Creatine, Vitamin D and Omega – 3 Supplement from Fish Oil. You might wonder if Omega 3 fatty acids from flax/chia seeds should be considered as well, but the fact is flax/chia seeds do not provide sufficient supplement on its own. Flax/chia seeds are found in the form of Alpha-Linoleic Acid (ALA) which has to be converted by the body into a usable form and the ratio conversion is rather poor.

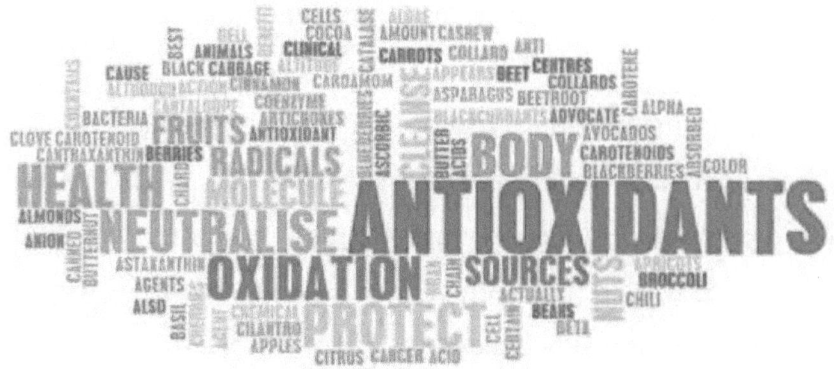

Diet Plan Tip: Foods are usually insufficient for anyone that is looking to gain muscles in the fastest manner, the best option is to take in the right supplements for your body needs.

Top 3 Muscle Gaining Supplements

Creatine / Creatine monohydrate

This is by far my top performance supplement for muscle gains.

Creatine monohydrate is by far the most tried and true, most affordable, and effective of all the creatine variants. It is original, and many subsequent variants of creatine are either inferior or cost more without giving any additional benefit. So creatine monohydrate is the specific type that I recommend, instead of those packed with additional glucose or unnecessary 'proprietary blend' (Most likely another marketing gimmick to inflate the price).

We get most of our creatine from animal products, mostly in meat, and it is more abundant in raw meat. When meat is cooked it degrades the creatine content, which is why it is difficult to get the performance-enhancing benefits without consuming this as a supplement.

To get creatine stores up to levels where they can benefit strength, power production, muscle fullness and ultimately your long-term ability to produce more muscle mass over time, I would recommend ingesting 0.018 g/lb of bodyweight per day (0.04 g/kg/ day). It will take a couple weeks of ingesting this amount per day to reach supplemental creatine levels, but after that point, you can just maintain those levels by continuing to take the dose, like the topping of your gas tank.

And last but not least, it's important to note that for long-term consumption, timing doesn't matter. It doesn't need to be taken with carbs, it doesn't need to be loaded, it doesn't need to be taken pre-workout, and it doesn't need to be taken post workout. All the benefits associated with creatine timing, whether it's taken with carbs, or if creatine is loaded in large amounts, are strictly related to the first couple weeks of consumption where the goal is to get to supplemental levels. It has nothing to do with long-term use and whether it takes you 5 days or 21 days to reach supplemental levels of creatine has a less than negligible effect on long-term gains. So, just take the daily dose I recommend and you'll be all set to reap its benefits.

Diet Plan Tip: It is best to consume Creatine after a workout but generally you can take it anytime. Moreover, it best not to take in Caffeine and Creatine at the same time as the effects may possibly counteract each other.

Vitamin D

Vitamin D is primarily produced in our body as a result of direct contact with sunlight. Having insufficient levels of vitamin D in the body can compromise the immune system, which can be a disaster for someone who is training hard, dieting or attempting to perform any type of activity at a high level.

Vitamin D also affects our mood and hormonal level. Furthermore, it's frequently linked to depression and psychological breakdown.

Vitamin D deficiency rates are a lot higher than we think, and being deficient in vitamin D can have negative impacts on muscular performance, immune function and hormonal status.

Thus, it's a good idea to supplement accordingly if you don't get much direct sunlight, have dark skin or a combination thereof. A basic dosing recommendation would be to take anywhere from 9-36 IU/lb/day (20-80 IU/kg/day) of vitamin D3 based on sunlight exposure. For those who find supplements that don't list the amount of Vitamin D3 in IU's, the equivalent dose in micrograms is 0.225 to 0.900 mcg/lbs/day (0.5 to 2 mcg/kg/day).

So if you work or train outdoors on a daily basis, you might not benefit from supplemental vitamin D3 at all. Perhaps taking 9 IU/lb (20 IU/kg) at most to be extra safe that you're getting enough would be a good idea. If you are someone on the opposite extreme end of the sunlight exposure spectrum, it might be more appropriate to take the full 36 IU/lb (80 IU/kg). So, you can regularly make sure to supplement the maximal effective dose throughout the winter, and in the summer months stop taking Vitamin D supplements.

If possible, the absolute best route would be to get your blood work checked to see where your levels are and to see if you're deficient. Otherwise, just use your best estimate in the range provided based on lifestyle and exposure to sunlight.

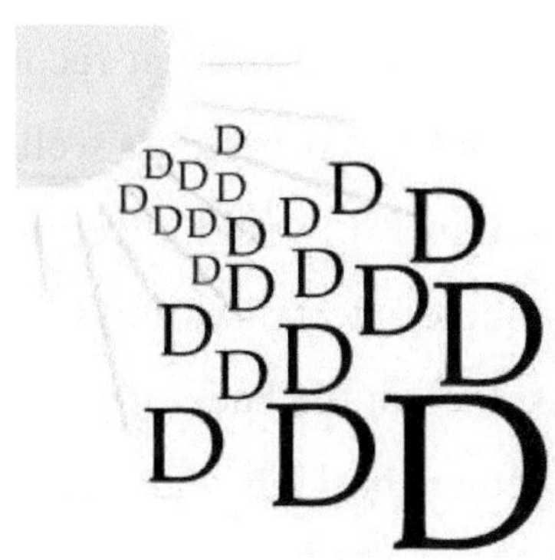

Supplement Facts: Vitamin D deficiency is relatively common in athletes and is associated with muscle weakness and atrophy, specifically Type 2 muscle fiber atrophy. Skipping out on this vitamin is just as bad as skipping out on leg day.

Fish Oil

Of the essential fatty acids (EFA's), eicosapentaenoic acid (EPA) and docosahexaenoic acid (DHA), which typically come from fish oil supplementation, have been found to have a host of potential health benefits. If you don't eat fish or don't like taking fish oil, you can also get EPA and DHA from an algae supplement, which is what the fish eat that gives them the EPA and DHA that we are looking for.

When appropriately dosed, EFA's help with leptin signaling in the brain, reducing inflammation, enhancing mood and reducing disease factor risk. They can also aid in joint recovery and have shown potential for some metabolic benefits as well.

Both while cutting or lean gaining, I would recommend getting enough EPA and DHA (combined) to fall within the 2 to 3 gram range per day. To check this, look at the back of your fish oil (or algae oil) container, add together the EPA and DHA and look at the serving size. Perhaps the label says that there is 400 mg per serving of EPA and DHA when combined. This would mean that you need 5 servings to get 2 grams (There is 1000 mg per gram).

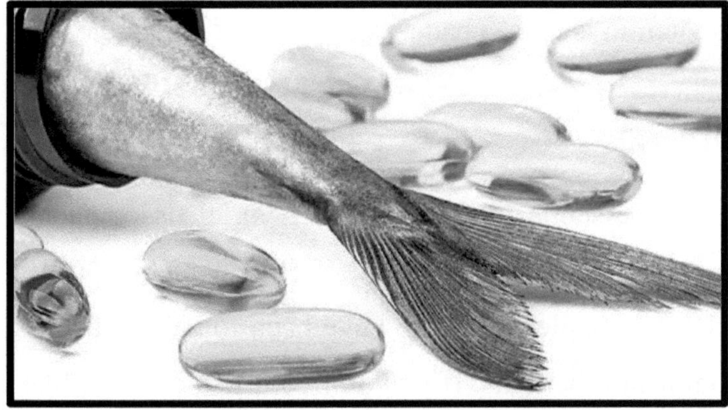

Supplement Facts: Fish oil can reduce blood clotting and should be supplemented with caution if blood-thinning medications, aspirin, warfarin or clopidogrel are already present in the body.

Rule of Thumb for a Good Diet

A good diet supposed to be simple and not to over-complicate things. Because the key to a sustainable fitness lifestyle is to have your diet simplified so that you're able to stick to it long-term.

For those who seek to gain muscles, your priority is not food restrictions. Instead, you should be focusing on the number of calories you're going to take throughout the day.

For starters, I recommend tracking your daily calories intake to havea clear picture of how your diet looks like and how you can manipulate it afterward.

Next is to determine what are your macronutrients percentage and finally the essential micronutrients (which can be easily covered with supplements).

Trust me, by becoming aware of your daily food intake, you will ultimately make better food choices in near future.

Diet Plan Tip: Preparation is the key to eating healthy. It may sound tricky and complex to prepare. Do not over-think it, instead choose foods that you enjoy eating and make a balanced meal.

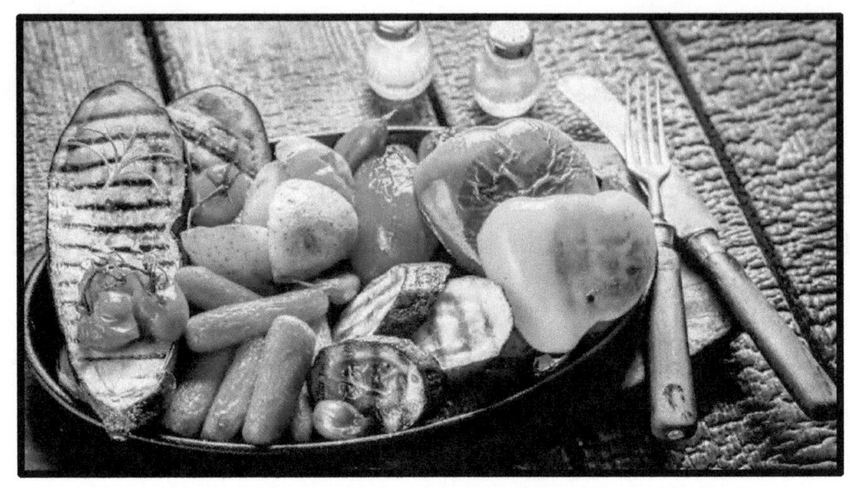

Foods to avoid

Generally, you should be avoiding food that makes you feel 'bloated', 'sick' and 'low-energy'. This includes processed, highly-toxic (with chemicals), junk food and sugary foods. Sugar is the main factor that you should really look out for as it is present in foods particularly that aren't fresh, frozen or dried. Additionally, sauces such as pasta sauce, ketchupand chili sauce contain sugar as well. Moreover, fruit juices and fizzy drinks are things that you need to avoid as well.

Supplements To Avoid

Supplements today are expensive! And if you're not careful, you'll end up burning a hole in your wallet with supplements that do not work.

There are a lot of people these days sold to the craze of muscle enhancing supplements that promise jaw-dropping muscle mass development. But honestly, do they even work? There are various supplements that that would improve muscle growth but only handful of it are actually scientifically proven to work if consume in the recommended method. Supplements that does not offer any muscle growth are considered placebo pills and powders which is merely an implication to your mind that it affects your body.

Supplements that develops placebo effect
1) Cyclotren
2) Clenbuterex
3) D-Pol
4) T-Bomb
5) Beastdrol
6) Somnidren

Testosterone Booster

They are supplements that increase testosterone levels in the blood, most of the compounds do boost testosterone levels and there are those which do not actually boost testosterone. It is recommended to cycle testosterone boosters as they do have side-effects that could be detrimental to your health if taken excessively.

Studies show that testosterone booster can actually cause testicles atrophy and lower HPTA stimulation if used excessively or with prolonged usage.

Also, it is shown that some even developed "adrenal fatigue" due to the chemical compounds in boosters.

There are 3 prime examples of compounds that have been scientifically proven that does not affect testosterone levels which are Tribulus Terrestris, ZMA, and D-aspartic acid.

- Tribulus Terrestris simply does not have any factors that would increase testosterone levels as well as body composition and improving exercise performance.

- ZMA is a combination of zinc, magnesium and vitamin B6 which is in the same line with Tribulus Terrestris. People who are deficient from zinc and magnesium would benefit their overall health but not for increasing testosterone level. The least ZMA could do is removing micronutrient deficiency that is suppressing testosterone production.

- D-aspartic acid could increase testosterone levels but the effects are short-lived and temporary, you could put into word it is unreliable.

There are various scientific studies that have been conducted to determine if increasing testosterone levels could help with boosting muscle gains. The results pretty much show that no matter how high you increase your testosterone levels, it would not help boost muscle building compared to consuming proper diet meals and viable supplements.

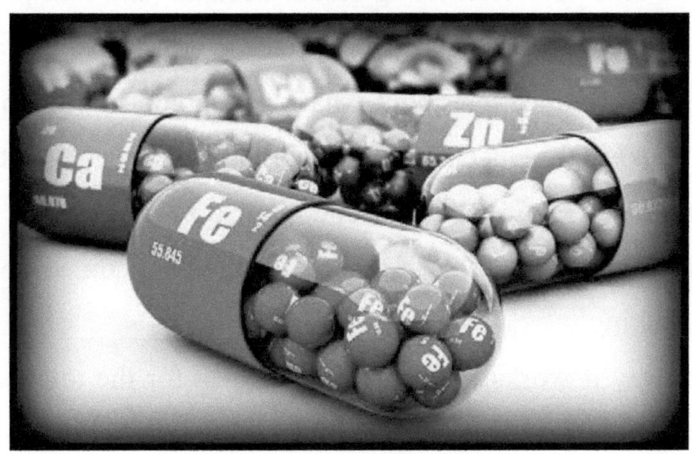

The key to building muscle is proper training and nutrition not reliance on supplements.

Protein Supplement Scams

We like protein powder. It's a quick, convenient and cost-effective way to hit our daily protein targets. Whey protein is not the cheapest, but it is popular due to the high BCAA content, particularly leucine, which is critical to the muscle building process.

Now, with consumers becoming wiser there is a rising demand for products that claim to have been lab tested, but this comes at a time of overall rising global demand (and thus prices). With consumers becoming sensitive to these price increases and a lack of general education about what they should be looking for on the packet, the incentives for companies to cut costs by cheating the system are all there, and many do.

I'm talking about the rise of the phenomenon known as 'protein spiking'.

The way it works is this: some labs test for the total amino acid content rather than the amounts of the individual amino acids themselves. This means that protein companies can dump cheap amino acids into the mix (mainly glycine and taurine), skimping on the actual whey content, which is expensive, and yet still pass some quality tests.

Here are some red flags to look out for when choosing a whey powder:

1. The cost per pound / kilo of claimed protein content is considerably cheaper than average. Whey is a commodity traded on the open market. You can be ripped off and pay way too much (You can even find places that sell 10x market price in luxury gyms!)

2. It has a proprietary blend (or doesn't list leucine content).

3. Leucine content, when listed, is lower than 2.7 g per 25 g of protein content (the BCAA content of whey is 25%, leucine should be 11%).

If your protein powder doesn't pass those checks, you're rolling the dice with the quality of what you're getting.

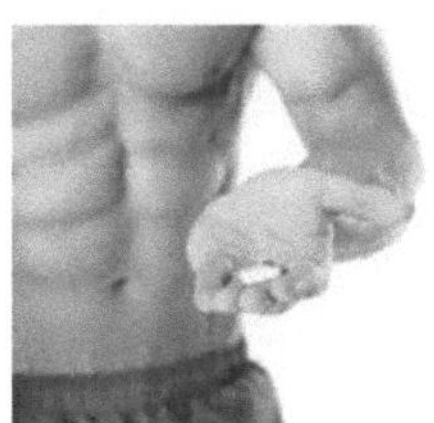

Protein supplement consumption is entirely optional and is based on personal preference. You can still opt for dieting instead of taking in protein powder.

Keeping in mind how adamant I am regarding the combined quality, validity and effectiveness of any substance, these are the supplements I highly recommend to everyone and especially useful for those of us interested in gaining muscle and strength.

Of course, there are other useful supplements worth mentioning such as Multivitamin, BCAA, HMB, Beta-alanine, glucosamine etc.

Now there's always some subjectivity in deciding whether these supplements are worth being on this list or not and as with all of my advice, feel free to disagree with it based on your own judgment. Additionally, it is quite likely that this list will prove to be outdated in a few years as more research comes out.

MUSCLE GAIN SECRETS 4

ULTIMATE CHEST & BEST
BICEPS SCULPTURING WORKOUTS

I'll share with you the ultimate chest & best biceps sculpturing workouts. These muscles groups will give you the V-figure that you've been longing for and look good in any outfit! So we're going to focus on that today, and we'll walk you through how to execute each workout with the perfect form to ensure maximal muscle growth and minimal injury.

First, we shall start off from one of the largest muscle groups of the body, apart from your legs and back – The Chest Muscles. The 3 most common ultimate chest workouts are:

1) Standard push-ups

2) Alternating one-handed push-ups

3) Shoulder adduction

1) Standard Push Ups

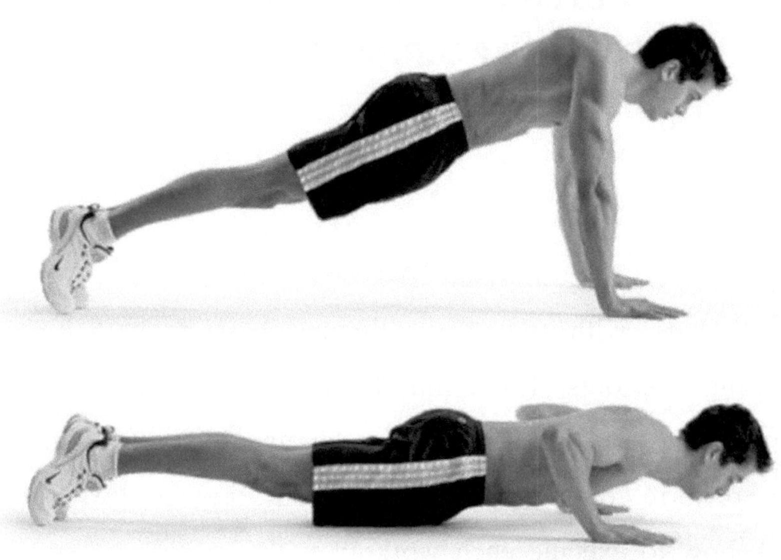

The standard push-up variation is best for beginners to develop overall pectoral muscles and if it's too difficult for you, go ahead and do knees push-ups – a variation where you place your knees while doing push-ups.

When you can do at least 30 push-ups and ready to move on to the advanced level, you can switch it up with different push-up variations to challenge yourself and engage different parts of your chest in building that full, nasty pecs!

1. Begin in the "up" position. Hand position can vary but should be at least slightly wider than the shoulders.

2. Keep the elbows close to your body and lower yourself very slowly.

3. Keep your back straight and do not allow the knees to touch the floor

4. Lower to within 1-2 inches of the floor and pause momentarily. Keeping your back straight, slowly raise your body to the "up" position.

5. Do not hold your breath. Practice inhaling and exhaling throughout the entire movement back and forth.

6. Do note that the wider your hand placement are, the more engagement will be involvedin the outer pectoral muscles.

2) Alternating One-Handed Push Up

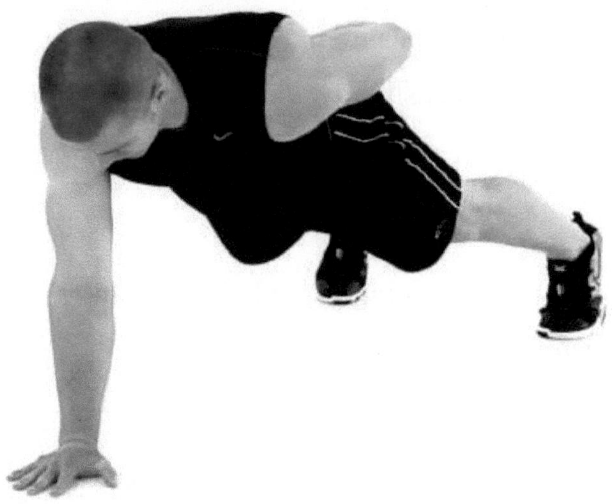

Want to challenge yourself to do something crazy? Try Alternating One-Handed Push Ups. And here's how you do it:

1. Spread your feet apart (Recommended as wide as your shoulder width for stability).

2. The active hand should be placed on the floor while the other hand can be placed behind the back.

3. This movement requires both stability and strength.

4. Just like doingnormal push-ups, you perform this exercise in a 2-point movement: Concentric motion during push,

and eccentric motion when you move back to the bottom in a slow and controlled manner. The only rule is not that you shouldn't touch the floor with your chest and knees. If it's too difficult for now, you can try doing this with knees on the ground.

3) Shoulder Adduction

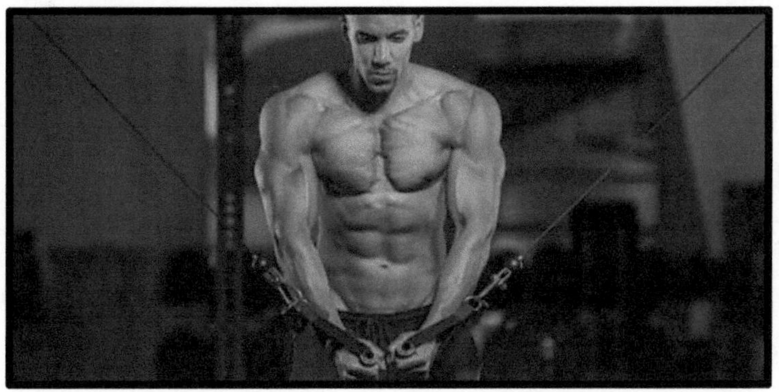

Another Ultimate Chest Workout that everyone should include into their routine is Shoulder Adduction or more commonly known as Chest Flys. Unlike push-ups and bench presses, Chest Fly workout engage the chest muscles more because this is a pure bodybuilding workout to sculpt the chest muscles; whereas bench press is more of a powerlifting workout.

And the range of motion of doing chest fly is a lot wider than presses. So how do you do it? Here's how you do a standard shoulder adduction:

1. Feet should be placed comfortably on the floor, making it easy to push against the ground for stability. (A seat belt helps to reduce excess body movement and isolate and exercise the chest muscles). The upper arms should be in line with the shoulders.

2. Begin with the upper arms parallel to the floor and outstretched to the side midline to the body, or behind the midline for a better stretch.

3. Bring the forearms together in a controlled movement. Do not slam the two pads into each other. The arms naturally tend to drop slightly as the forearms are brought together.

4. Allow the forearm pads to return slowly to their starting position

5. Breathing techniques can vary, but you should either inhale or exhale on each movement. Many individuals find it easier to exhale on the concentric contraction of bringing the forearms together and then inhale on the eccentric contraction of returning to the start position. Do not squeeze your hand grip because this detracts from the workout of the chest muscles by using extra energy.

This is one common variation. Most people like using cable for adduction or flys, but you can also use dumbbells or even kettlebells. Some prefer standing, while some prefer to do it while laying on a bench. You can always switch things up for more variation because variety is the spice of life! You don't want your workout to be a boring routine, so make sure to keep things fun and interesting.

Honestly, the 3 workouts that I mentioned earlier can really help you grow some awesome pectoral muscles especially if you're a beginner. A simple routine with 4 Sets of the 3 Workouts can ensure optimal muscle growth because they engaged different angles of the muscles. For more advanced lifters, here are some additional chest workouts:

1. Barbell bench press
2. Incline bench press
3. Dumbbell bench press
4. Close-grip bench press

1) Barbell Bench Press

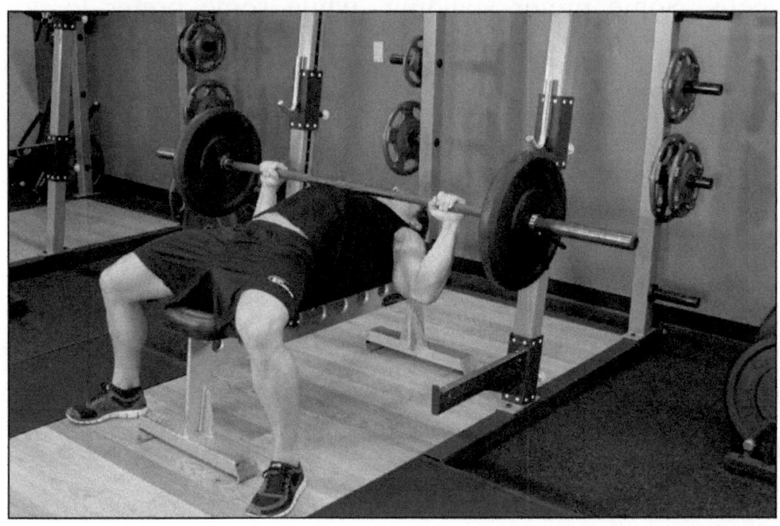

Presses are more of a power movement and require proper understanding of each movement and perform with the right form as injuries are very common in presses. The most common reasons of injury in presses are carrying too much weight and improper form of execution. So how do you properly execute Chest Press movements?

Number 1- Barbell Bench Press

1.   Make sure to lie in a comfortable position on the bench to ensure safety and powerful execution. Usually, your eyes are beneath the bar at the starting position.

2.   Before you begin execution, make sure to arch your back slightly to bring those shoulder blades together and always keep your chest up.

3.   Hand placement on the bar is totally up to you, and you can manipulate hand movement for different variations of bench press such as standard bench press, wide-grip bench press, close-grip bench press and underhand bench press.

4.   To execute bench press properly with maximal power output, make sure to plant your feet firm on the ground because you should be utilizing leg drive in this movement.

5.   Unrack the weight carefully and perform the movement in horizontal movement until it touches your chest, then execute full power to push the bar upwards. Repeat this movement until the repetitions have been completed.

Remember to squeeze your shoulder blades together when you perform Bench Presses and tuck your elbows in at 45 degrees angle for safety and proper execution. A lot of guys risk screwing up their elbows and shoulder joints for not following these 2 simple tips.

Also, start light and drop your ego in the gym. Ego-lifting is a surefire way to the hospital and if you don't want to suffer from unnecessary pain and injuries, be honest with yourself and pick the weight you can handle. Your only goal is to make progress in your fitness goal and not impress others in the gym.

2) Incline Bench Press

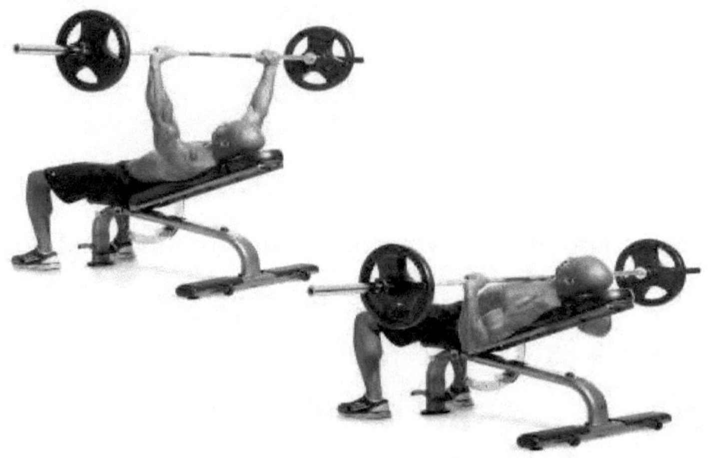

As mentioned before, the chest muscles are made up of different parts and angles. The common ones are the Upper chest and the Lower chest; The Outer, Middle and Inner Chest. The upper chest is the least developed part of the majority and you should really focus on this part more as the upper chest provides the illusion of you having fuller and mightier pecs. And the best workout to target the upper chest is the Incline Bench Press.

1. Don't attempt to lift weights that are too heavy for you at the moment. Otherwise, you might risk breaking your wrist or neck if you're not careful.

2. Again, lay flat on the bench and plant your feet firm on the ground. You should be utilizing leg drive in pressing motion. Retract your scapula with a slight arch and lock into this position. Now, you're good to go.

3. Grip the bar firmly and unrack when you're ready. You can easily unrack the barbell by simply extending your arms straight. Now, you're at the starting position to execute the full movement.

4. One thing to take note of is to perform this exercise in a controlled manner, you don't want to swing around heavy weights and injure yourself. Slowly lower the bar to your chest with your elbows tucked in. Keep your body tight throughout the entire exercise and remember to utilize leg drive.

5. At the bottom of the movement, push the bar back up to the starting position with the powerful concentric pushing

motion. Repeatm this movement until your rep scheme has been completed.

3) Dumbbell Bench Press

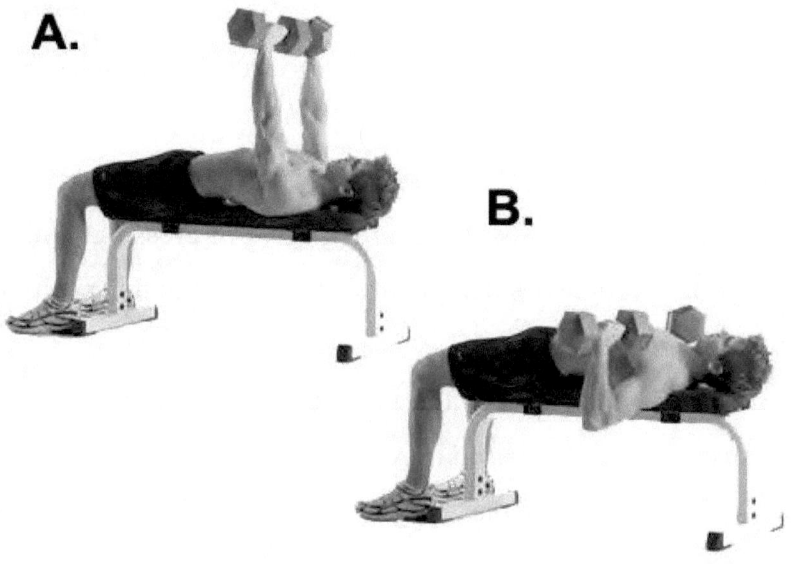

This can be said to be a more advanced level of push-ups as it engages the chest more and you're able to make progress with heavier weights. Here's how you perform Dumbbell Bench Press properly:

1. First, find 2 dumbbells which are suitable for you to execute dumbbell bench press properly. Not too light and not too heavy, enough to execute 8-10 reps before failure is the sweet spot. Next, sit on a flat bench with dumbbells in both hands on your side, resting on your thighs.

2. Then, you can easily get into position by using your thighs to raise those dumbbells to your side at shoulder width.

3. Once at shoulder width, the dumbbells should be just to the sides of your chest. Remember to protract your shoulder blades and you should form a 45-degree angle at your armpit. This will be the bottom of your lift.

4. Now is the time to execute the concentric motion. Remember to keep your body tight at all times and exhale when you push. Just like performing barbell bench press, you can use leg drive for more power. Remember to squeeze your pecs at the top of the lift. Then slowly lower your dumbbells to the bottom position in a slow tempo.

5. Repeat the exercise until your rep scheme has been completed.

4) Close-Grip Bench Press

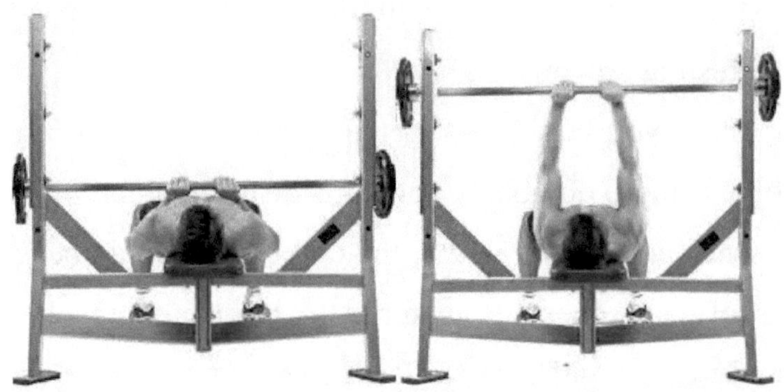

This workout focuses on the Inner Pecs and Triceps.

1. The starting position is the same as performing the normal bench press. The only difference in this lift is the hand position, which you'll be placing your hands close together firmly on a barbell (your grip can be supinated or pronated in this lift). Carefully unrack the barbell and lock into this starting position.

2. Slowly lower the barbell to your chest with your elbows tuck in. You will feel more burn in your triceps in this lift because close-grip bench press involves more triceps activation.

3. From the bottom of the lift, push the bar back up to the starting position with one clean, powerful motion. You will feel

tightness in both your chest and triceps as you move the bar upwards. After that, slowly lower the bar once again at a slower tempo.

4. Repeat this movement until your rep scheme has been completed.

5. Finally, rack the bar after you're done with the exercise.

Best Biceps Sculpturing Workouts

Biceps are the epitome of fitness. Every man and woman deserves to have some awesome biceps. So you should really incorporate biceps workouts into your routine to grow these proud muscles. And here are my best biceps sculpturing workouts.

1) Standing barbell curl
2) Ez-bar preacher curl
3) Alternate incline dumbbell curl
4) Reverse wrist curl and wrist curl
5) Seated barbell curl
6) Dual dumbbell hammer curl

1) Standing Barbell Curl

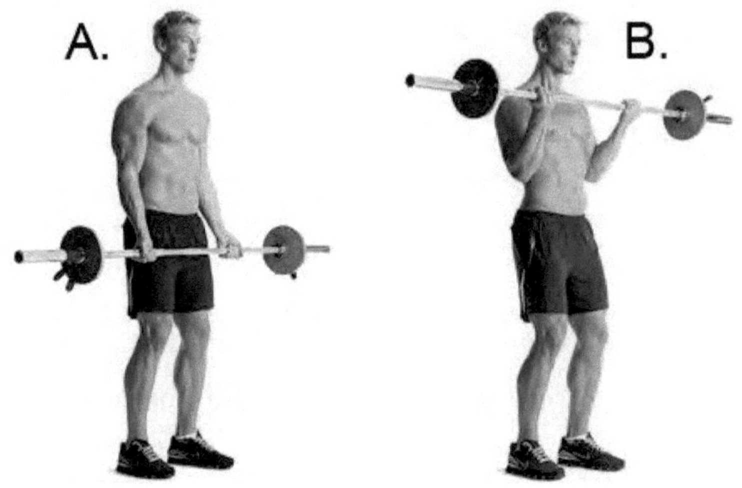

Standing Barbell Curl – The most basic biceps workout you can see in any posters and magazines. Engages both your total biceps at the same time.

1. Do not go overboard with biceps curls as you may tear your biceps tendon if you're not careful - So only pick weights that you can handle. Then, grasp the barbell at shoulder-width apart with palms facing upwards.

2. Stand tall upright with knees slightly bent to buffer the weight during exercise. Allow the bar to hang to your thighs and this will be your starting position.

3. In order to execute the exercise flawlessly, slowly curl the bar in a controlled tempo and squeeze at the top of the lift. You can definitely feel the pump in your biceps as your squeeze at the top.

4. After squeezing your biceps at the top, slowly lower the bar back to the starting position in slow eccentric motion.

5. Repeat this movement and remember not to cheat your way through by swinging with unwanted momentum. You want to make sure you always keep the tension on in order to get the most out of this exercise.

2) EZ-Bar Preacher Curl

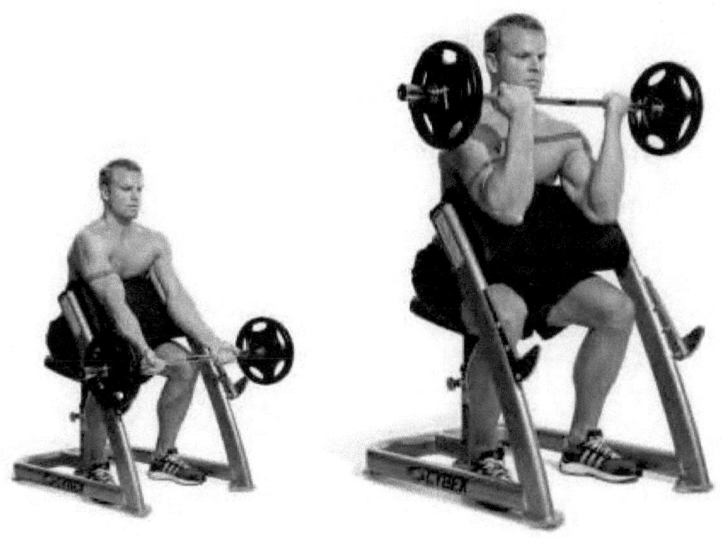

This workout engages your inner biceps and brings out the biceps peak.

1. Look for a bicep curls station in order to perform this exercise. Firstly, adjust your seat height to a comfortable position so that your arms are properly rested on the pad. This will be your starting position.

2. For better stabilization, place your feet wide and frontward, and hold tight onto the EZ-bar with the supinated grip.

3. Perform the curls in a controlled manner and remember to squeeze at the top of the lift to reap the most benefits. Finally, lower the bar back to the starting position. Repeat this movement until your rep scheme has been completed.

3) Alternate Incline Dumbbell Curl

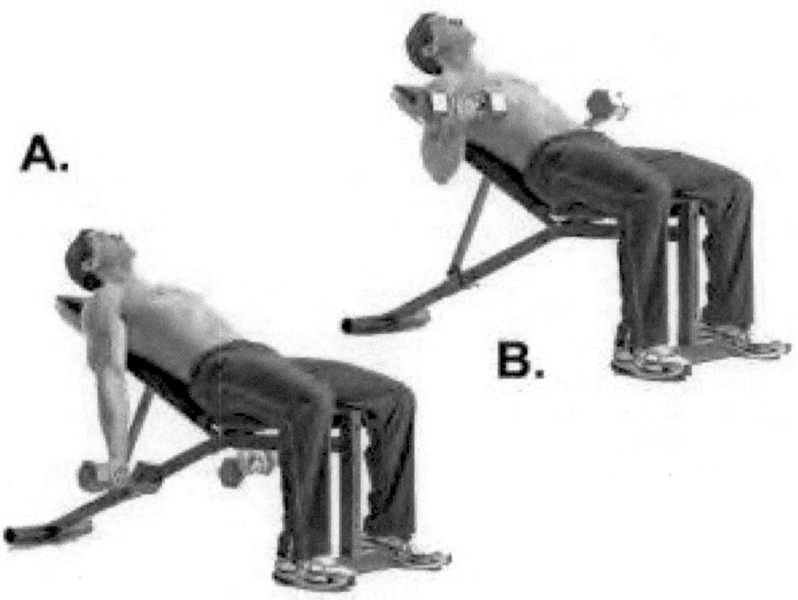

This is my favorite workout hands down because this workout is a perfect isolation workout for the biceps without any cheating movements – the incline position cancels out most of the 'cheating' momentum, increase the range or motion, and you can't really carry much weight when you're lying incline.

1. Set an incline bench at about a 45-degree angle.

2. Hold onto 2 dumbbells in both hands with a neutral grip and allow your arm to hang low. This will be the starting position.

3. Lock your elbows in this position to reduce cheating momentum. Slowly raise the dumbbell upwards (you can start with either side first) and add a little twist at the top while you squeeze the biceps.

4. Twist and squeeze your biceps at the top for 2-3 seconds before slowly lower the weights back to the starting position.

5. Once completed, repeat this movement with the other arm until your rep scheme has been completed.

I recommend doing 10-12 Reps for 3-4 sets for this exercise to effectively grow your biceps.

4) Reverse Wrist Curl And Wrist Curl

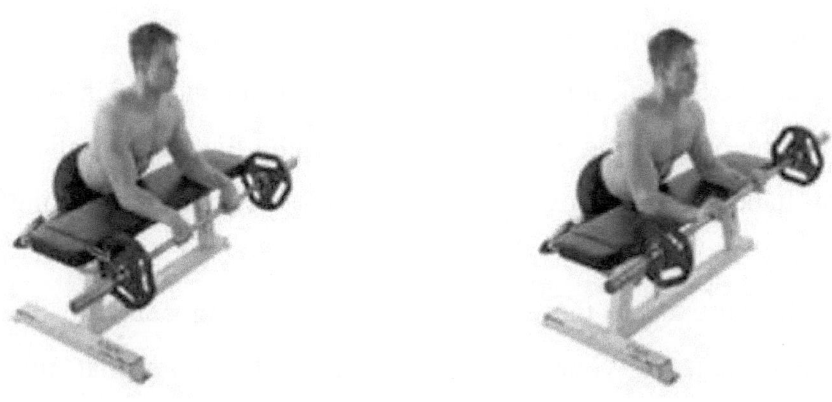

This additional workout trains your wrists and forearms. Many people ignore this exercise because they don't see the need of it. But do you want to look like a hunk with huge biceps and triceps with arms like twigs? If you want to look good overall and have strong stabilization muscles to move more weights, add in these 2 compulsory forearms workout into your workout regime.

1. You perform reverse wrist curls with a pronated grip (also known as the overhand grip). Make sure to pick a light weight for this exercise as your forearms are not huge muscles to handle massive weights.

2. Next, look for a bench and kneel at the side of it, with your forearms resting on the bench. Grasping the barbell, allow your hands to hang over the edge. This will be the starting position.

3. To execute the exercise, simply curl your hands to the top and squeeze your forearms muscles (Do note that this exercise has a short range of motion). Then, slowly lower the weight to the starting position.

4. Repeat this movement until your rep scheme has been completed.

Since the forearms have smaller muscles and shorter range or motion, you don't have to go too heavy on this. Simply lift lighter weights in higher repetition to get the best result from this exercise.

5) Seated Barbell Curl

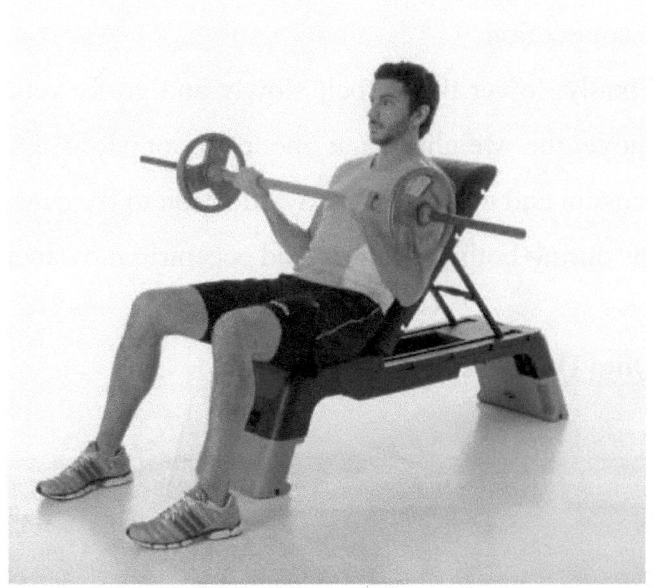

This is another variation for bicep curls. This exercise is similar to standing barbell curls. The only difference is you're seated this time round.

1. First, load up your barbell with appropriate weight to perform 6-10 reps max.

2. Sit upright on an adjustable bench and rest the barbell on your thighs.

3. With a supinated grip, perform curls in a control movement without swinging the weights around. Again, you want to make sure that you squeeze at the top of the lift and feel the biceps contraction.

4. Finally, lower the barbell slowly and go for repetitions. Always move the weights in a moderate or slow tempo for constant tension and contraction. Pay attention to the sensation of your biceps during both concentric and eccentric movements.

6) Dual Dumbbell Hammer Curl

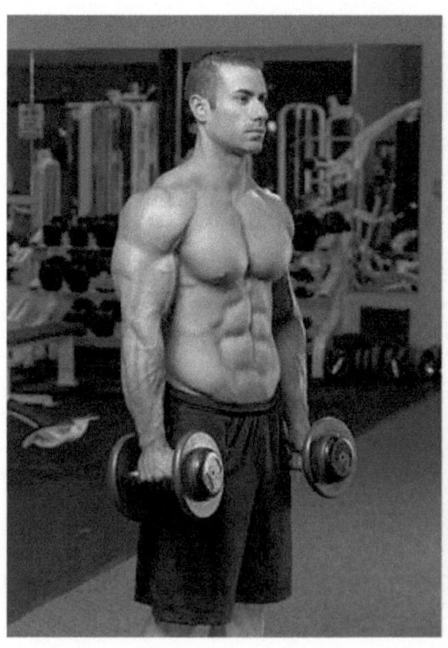
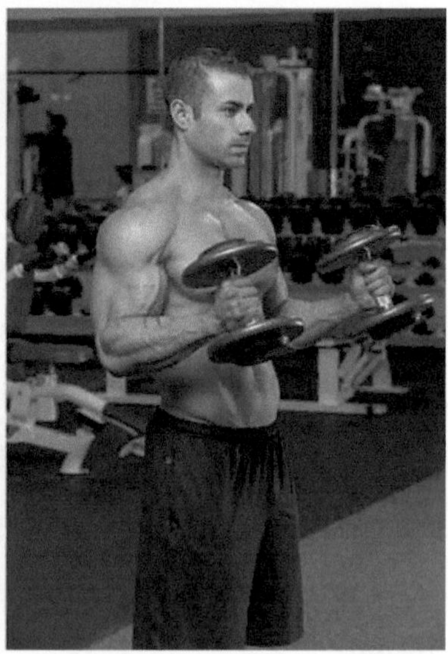

A killer workout for both forearms and biceps. Every biceps workout routine should have hammer curls in to be complete.

1. You can choose to stand or stay seated for this workout. First, grasp on tightly a pair of dumbbells by your side with a neutral grip. This will be your starting position.

2. Make sure that your palms are facing each other throughout the entire workout. Hammer curls require lifting both dumbbells in an upward motion in elbows-locked position without twisting your wrists.

3. Squeeze your biceps at the top of the lift and slowly return to the starting position by slow, controlled eccentric movement. Repeat this exercise until you've completed your reps.

So there you have it, ultimate chest and biceps sculpturing workouts you can add to your workout routine and grow those highly esteemed muscles!

HOW TO GET "THE ROCK" SHOULDER

Everyone wants to have "The Rock" shoulder & Washboard Abs! These are the aesthetic muscles that make you look good with or without clothes.

First, let's start off with "The Rock" Shoulders. Some even call it the "Diamond Delts" and even" The Boulders". Whatever you call it, round, rock-solid and striated shoulders are highly sought after by anyone who are into fitness.

So how do you get "The Rock" Shoulder? Essentially there are 3 angles you need to tackle to have round, solid deltoids or 'delts', which are: Front Delts, Middle Delts, and Rear Delts. Here are my simplified and complete workouts to fully engage every angle of your delts in making them pop:

1) Lateral shoulder raise

2) Standing side deltoid circle raise

3) Seated overhead military press

4) Seated alternated dumbbell press

5) Upright rowing

6) Seated bent-over rear deltoid raise

1) **Lateral Shoulder Raise**

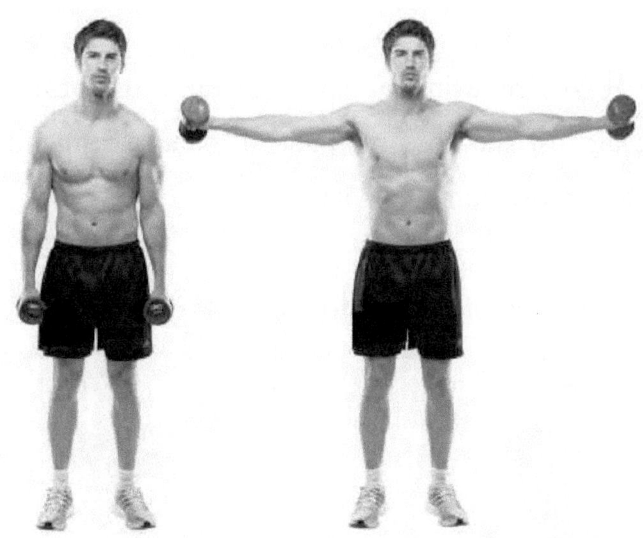

Lateral Shoulder Raise, the best lateral deltoid exercise in history. This is the best exercise to sculpt round shoulders and giving others the impression of you having huge and wide shoulders.

1. Position the height of the seat so that the feet are firmly planted on the floor. This gives resistance against the floor and assists in balance and stability while lifting. The seat should be adjusted to a comfortable position to perform the movement.

2. Depends on the type equipment you use – whether it's Dumbbell or Lateral Raise Machine, you either place the forearms against the pads or grip the handles. Start with your arms at your sides.

3. If you're using a machine, raise the arms up while pushing against the forearm pads. If you're using dumbbells, simply raise those dumbbells laterally.

2) Standing Side Deltoid Circle Raise

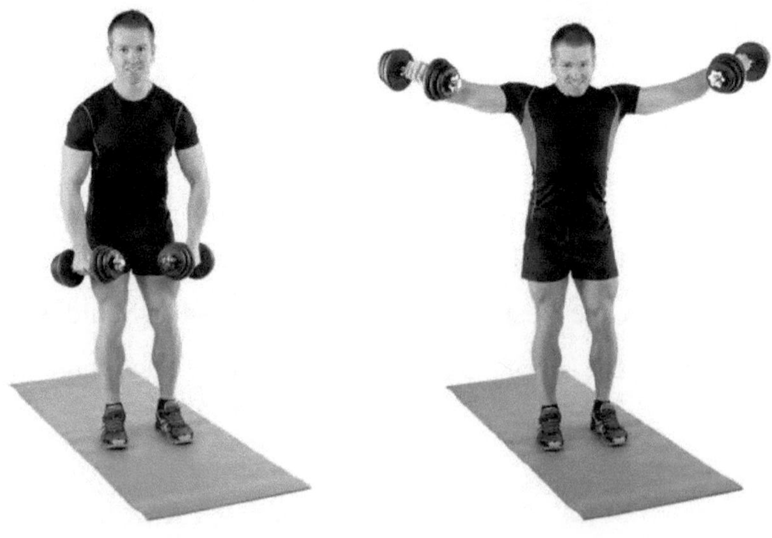

Standing Side Deltoid Circle Raise, one of the best exercise for overall shoulder muscles development in all different angles.

1. Pick up the weights with your palms facing each other. Try to use your legs to lift the weight, rather than your back. Keep the back straight and the head up.

2. Stand up straight with your feet positioned in a comfortable stance so you are well balanced and relaxed. The feet should be about shoulder-width apart; the arms should be fully extended at your sides with a dumbbell in each hand.

3. You begin with both dumbbells hang on your side. At the same time, raise both dumbbells out to the sides, bringing them up just above shoulder height. It is acceptable to flex the elbows slightly as the weights are brought up.

4. Lower the weights using the same lateral motion with which they were raised.

Usually, you can't go heavy on this exercise. So take a light weight and perform 8-10 circles of each set of this exercise.

3) Seated Overhead Military Press

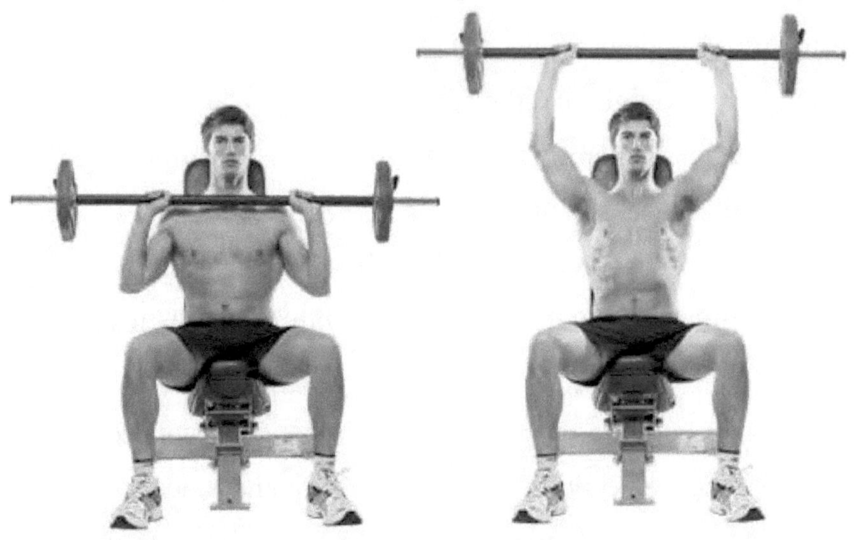

Seated Overhead Military Press, a power movement to develop the mid deltoids.

1. You can perform military press using dumbbells, kettlebells or barbell. First, make sure to sit upright on a stool. Grasp onto your barbell with shoulder-width apart.

2. At the starting position, both of your elbows are tucked in and the bar lay on your upper chest. To execute the movement, simply push the bar upward with your arms fully extended. The bar or dumbbells should be at the overhead position at the top of the lift.

3. One thing you need to make sure is to keep your core tight, spine erect and head held up as you perform the exercise.

4. Finally, lower your weights slowly until its back to the starting position. You don't want the weight slamming down at you so make sure you move the weights in a slow, controlled tempo for gains and safety.

4) Seated Alternated Dumbbell Press

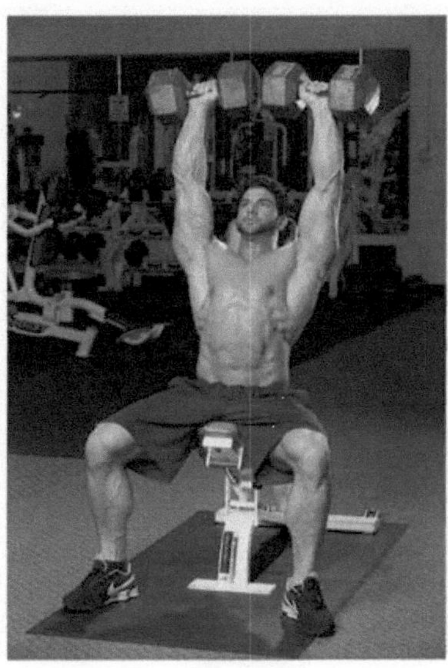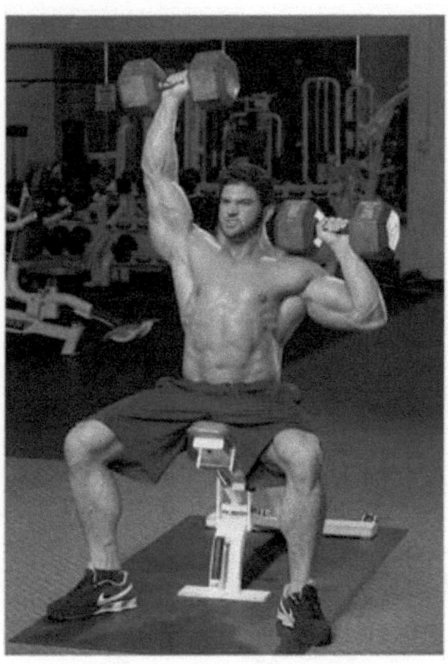

Seated Alternated Dumbbell Press, another variation of military press with more control and isolation.

1. Lift two dumbbells in a continuous motion, keeping the back straight and the head up, until they are at shoulder height.

2. Position the feet firmly on the floor and push against the floor for stability. Notice that the heel of the prosthetic leg is pushing against the floor.

3. Keep the elbows out to the sides and the thumbs facing each other.

4. Lift to mid-chest level.

5) Upright Rowing

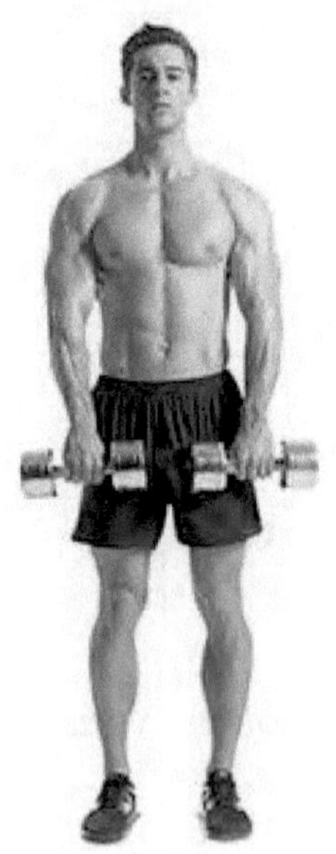
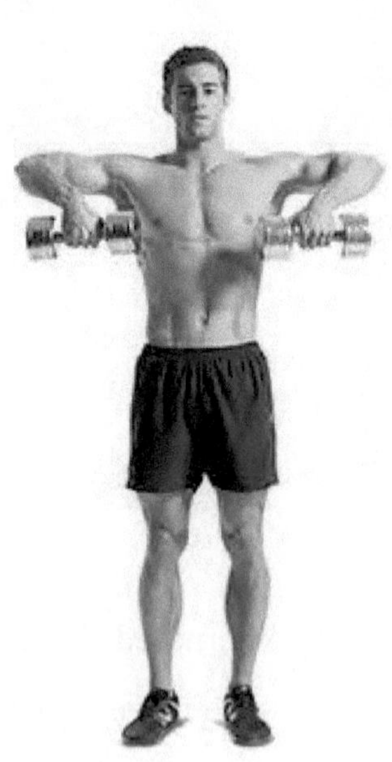

Upright Rows, a killer workout for the middle deltoids.

1. First, stand upright with your knees slightly bent to buffer the weights. Then, prepare a set of dumbbells, kettlebells, barbell or EZ-barbell to perform the exercise.

2. To move into the starting position, stand upright with the weights hanging on both sides.

3. Your feet should be shoulder-width apart and slightly bent for balance.

4. You should apply overhand grip for this exercise and keep both hands close to each other. From that position, raise the weights upward to your chin in a pulling motion. Imagine carrying 2 pails of water vertically while standing upright.

5. At the top of the lift, the elbows should flare out to the sides and keep them as high as possible.

6. Remember to pause and squeeze at the top of the lift before lowering them back down to the startingposition.

7. Repeat the movement until you've completed your desired repetitions.

6) Seated Bent-Over Rear Deltoid Raise

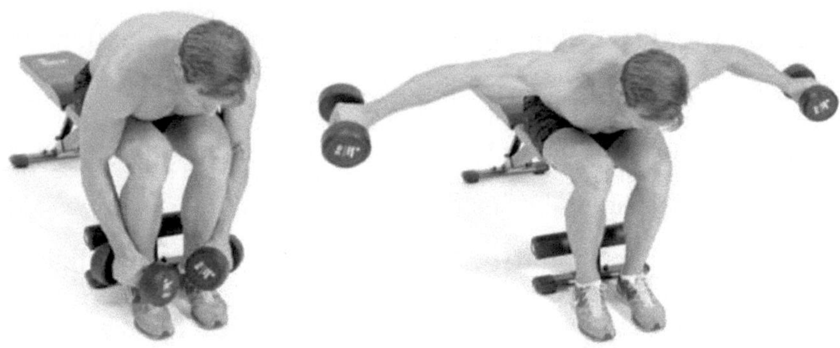

This workout targets the rear delts, a part where most people neglect but essential to bring out the round, boulders. Here's how you do it:

1. Select two lightweight dumbbells (10 pounds or less for the beginner); place them on the floor on either side of the end of a flat bench.

2. Sit at the end of the bench with your feet fairly close together and planted firmly on the floor. The dumbbells should be on either side below where you are sitting.

3. Lean forward so that your chest almost touches your thighs. Keep your head facing the floor. Lift the dumbbells to the height of your ears.

4. Raise the dumbbells out and upward, straightening your arms and locking the elbows.

5. Lower and raise the dumbbells in a continuous semi-circular motion, keeping your arms straight and elbows locked.

6. Inhale as the dumbbells are raised; exhale as they are lowered.

You don't have to go heavy for this exercise, as the rear delts are not huge muscles. Try doing it for 12-15 reps each set with control for best results.

How To Get Washboard Abs

Are you slumping in the couch right now? With your tummy bulging from beneath your shirt? Fatty, one pack, beer belly - are you sick and tired of these words?

Or have you been suffering from being overly skinny and bony, that it makes you feel small, weak and vulnerable?

Abs is a short form for abdominal, which is your stomach muscles.

A well-developed rectus abdominis or six-pack abs, seems to be the end goal of any exercise regimen. It is this muscle group that is one of the most challenging to build, as tons of effort and brutally intense workout do not magically guarantee a successful outcome. Think of your abs as a bi-product, not a muscle that you build. Like a bonus of work from a job well done.

But if you aim for overall well-being first and six-pack abs second, you are more likely to keep up the vigorous training needed to get that enviable perfect physique.

The Solid Foundation To Get Washboard Abs

1. Burn Your Fats First

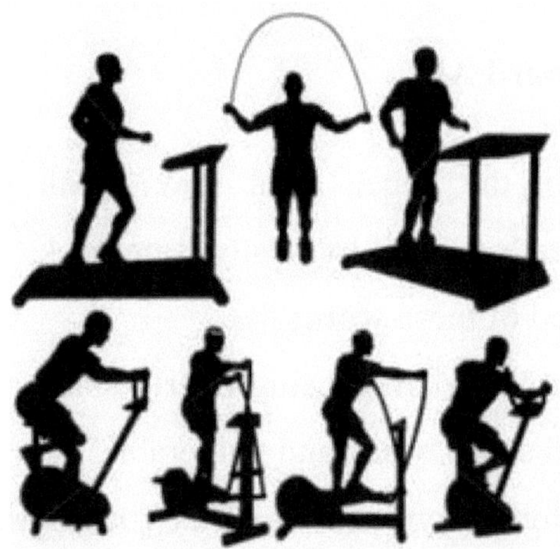

Want to burn those unwanted fats? Perform some regular aerobic activity. You can't spot-reduce abdominal fat. You need to burn your overall body fat before your body allows you to start building specific muscle group.

Cycling, jogging, running, jumping rope, and swimming are some good aerobic exercises to achieve this. To enable your body to begin burning your stored fat, you should blast fat for at least 30 minutes by performing heart-rate-elevating exercises. This is because your body only burns energy from food during the first 20 minutes. The ideal calculation is 30 minutes for at least four times a week. It is best done before breakfast as it triggers your body to burn your previously stored fats.

2. Crunches Exercise

Tone your abs with crunches. There are three types of crunches to target specific region of your abdominal area to achieve an evenly sculptured washboard abs.

- **Regular crunches (tones upper abdomen)**

1. Find a place with a solid support for your back. Lie on an exercise mat to prevent straining your back.

2. Your knees should be bent. Your feet position should be as wide as your hips and both should be flat on the floor. Your hands should be behind your head. Hold your chin forward, not

tucked into your chest. Try to gaze at ceiling while you're doing this workout to ensure your chin is in the right, safe position.

3. Exhale contract your abs muscle. Use your abs muscle to lift your head. Do not pull your head up with your hands.

4. Pause for a moment. Squeezing your abdominal muscle as you do so then inhale slowly and ease your back down the starting position. You must control your movement while lifting your back up and going back down. Do not release and let go rapidly.

5. Relax your muscles for a moment, exhale and repeat. Throughout the exercise, be mindful to keep your knees bent and your feet in the same position. Never lift your lower back off the floor.

- **Reverse crunches (tones lower abdomen)**

1. Similar to the regular crunch, your hands are behind your head, your shoulders off the floor, but this time you are going to have knees in the air to start the movement.

2. With your feet and knees up, pull your knees as close as you can and hold that position. From there just go back and forth

3. A good reverse crunch that targets the lower abs would be a small movement

4. Each crunch needs to be a squeeze and not a rocking motion

5. Don't let your upper body move too much.

6. Repeat for several times.

• Bicycle crunches (tones obliques, aka "love handles")

1. Find a place with a solid support for your back.

2. You can support your hands behind your head to make sure you are not yanking on your neck. This may cause pain and problems. You are just supporting your head.

3. Keep your shoulder blades off the ground. Bring knees up to 90 degrees. Bring your right elbow to left knee as you alternate side to side. Your goal is to get your elbow as close to the inside of that knee as you can

4. Now simultaneously, slowly go through a cycling motion

5. Continue alternating in this manner.

6. Bear in mind that it is essential that you increase the difficulty of your exercises and change the variety of your workout routines every two months. This is to allow your muscle to recuperate and burn calories efficiently. Do these routines at

least three times a week. Remember that crunches are best done very slowly and always with control.

3. Eat smart

Avoid processed foods (at all means if you can!). Foods that have undergone preservation or packing have lost their nutrients. And worse, processing adds on unhealthy fats, plenty of sugar or sugar substitute, and synthetic vitamins and minerals. Most the ingredients in processed foods include sweeteners, coloring, and hydrogenated oils. These ingredients are not even recognized by your body as edible ingredients, so they end up being stored as fats.

4. Eat healthy fats

Fats have a bad reputation, but not all fats are harmful. Dietary fats coming from monounsaturated and polyunsaturated fats are food for you. Olive oils, fish oils, natural peanut butter, avocado, and almonds are some really good examples.

Just make sure to keep your intake between 20% and 30% to regulate your calories. This will help stabilize your insulin level, which if too high, causes fat retention. By eating healthy fats, you are more likely to stay away from the fridge looking for food, as these healthy fats tend to keep you sated for a longer time. Most often, eating only protein or carbs alone will make you hungry more often.

5. Drink plenty of water

Studies have shown that people who drink a lot of water lose more weight and are able to keep it off longer. Adequate water intake boosts your metabolism rate. Drinking more water helps you stay away from empty-calorie drinks like soda and processed juice.

6. Eat good carbs

Good carbs like whole grains are rich in fiber and go through your system much slower than refined, white carbs. Therefore, it avoids spikes in blood sugar levels. Instead of your normal to-go carbs, always opt for healthy carbs – whole grains, nuts, pumpkin, potatoes.

7. Eat protein for breakfast

What's more important than feeling your tummy with protein early in the morning? A protein-packed breakfast is closely related to increased feelings of fullness and this would help to reduce your desire to snack. For example, instead of the usual ham and eggs, maybe you can go for nuts, egg whites, and cottage cheese. Eat less but often. Rather than eating 3 big meals per day, you can eat 5 meals per day, but each with a smaller portion. When your body in hungry, it likes to hoard fat, causing you to crave foods like pizza, burgers, and pastries. If you're rarely hungry, your metabolism learns to stabilize, and you won't feel food cravings.

If you would like to try a stricter diet to keep your blood sugar level balanced throughout the day, eat 4 - 5 proper meals in bite-sized portions. You tend to not overeat this way, because you'll be consuming foods high in fiber, protein and nutrients.

We've just unlocked the secrets to getting washboard abs! It's all about making small lifestyle choices in order to reduce body fat! Eat clean, take it easy on junk food, drink plenty of water work those abs and do cardio!

Abs are yours for the taking!

CELEBRITY WORKOUT

Adding Celebrity Exercise to your workout plan

Once your diet is all set and you're confident with what you can eat, it's time to put the workout into play. There are various types of workout you can choose, depending on your goals and what you like to do with your personal time. The most significant point is that you need to seek something that you enjoy doing or really want to do. It is not necessary to determine a certain type of workout because it's what you feel you are needed to do. There are various choices. If you think that this type of workout does not appeal to you, you can shift to a different workout.

When it comes to celebrity workout plans, they are barely an accurate representation of what the individual actually did. Most celebrity workout plans that you could find on the Internet would probably lack information about the individual's nutrition, recovery protocol and prior training history and so on. Most importantly, everyone's physique is built differently. Instead of relying on using a celebrity's ideal physique as a target to desire for, use them as inspiration to stay consistent with your training/diet. Genetics play a significant role in how a person's muscles are developed and shaped and no amount of workout will change how you are physiologically built.

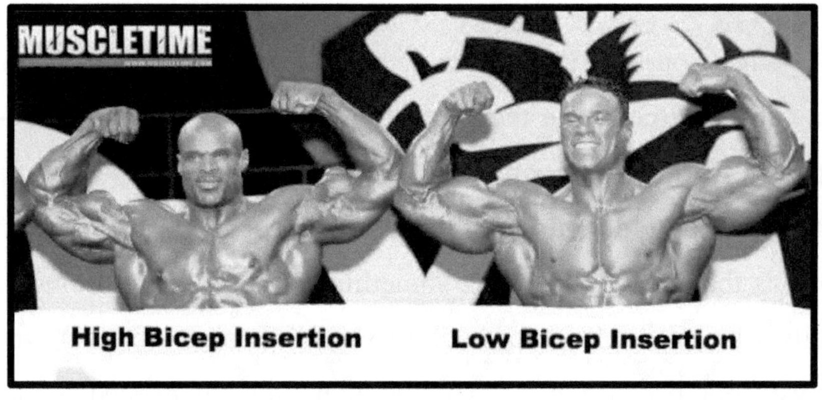

Differences between High/Low Bicep Insertions: Performing bicep curls will not change your insertions. Muscle Insertion affects all muscle on your body and biceps are a simple example to illustrate this point.

Practicing Celebrity Workouts

Personally, you can still follow your desired celebrity workout plan as a stepping stone to achieve your goals of muscle building. But in terms of diet plan, it is not ideal to straight-out follow their diet plans even if it is out there for people to look up to. Our daily caloric needs are varied from individual to another individual, even if you have the exact same weight and body metabolism doesn't expect to gain the same results as what they have achieved. Nonetheless, let's look into several celebrity workouts that shape into everyone desired body.

Daniel Craig

Famous for his role as the current James Bond 007 agent in the James Bond franchise film, he spent months to tune his body just for this particular role. He took on weight training 5 days a week followed by light cardio with stretching on the weekends, stayed consistent with the ideal diet plan and had a personal trainer and dietician to keep him in line. As he was not overweight prior to engaging in his workout, he just needed to lose a proper amount of weight and build muscles. Generally, most people would concentrate on one muscle group per day, working it only once a week, Daniel worked on full body circuits, boosting boosted his heart rate and developed muscle and endurance at the same time.

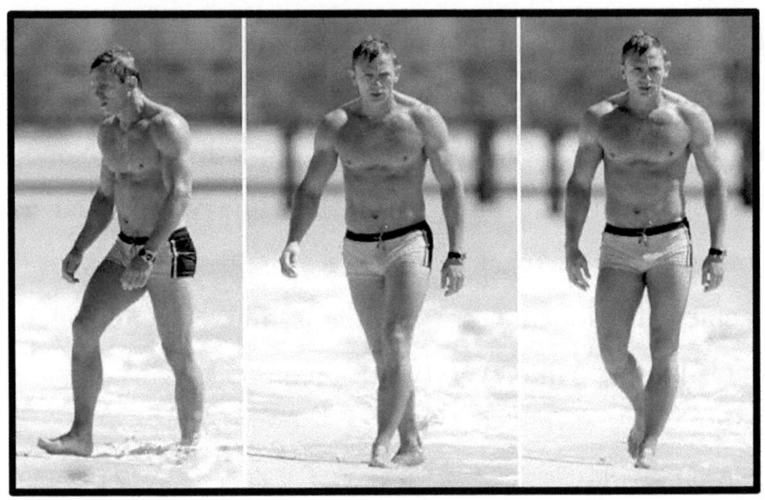

Daniel Craig physique back in James Bond:

Casino Royale (2006)

Full Body Circuit (Weekdays) with Light Cardio (Weekends)

A full body circuit is a workout that jumps from one exercise to another with minimal rest. This is the optimum way to build muscle and burn fat at the same time. Moreover, it is an effective workout in burning fat than a traditional cardio routine. On the weekdays he would be doing 10 reps of each exercise and move onto the next exercise and do 10 reps without rest until he completes the circuit. Moreover, he does it in 3 complete sets of the circuit, reducing rest time. The reasoning behind how he was able to conduct the workout back to back is because the workout encompasses various muscle groups. In this manner, your body will not overexert itself.

The following is Daniel Craig's workout plan:

1. Monday's Workout (Power Circuit 10 reps per exercise with 3 sets)
• Clean and Press
• Weighted Knee Raise
• Weighted Step-ups
• Pull ups
• Incline Push-up
• Triceps Dips

2. Tuesday's Workout (Chest & Back 10 reps per exercise with 4 sets)
• Incline Bench press
• Pull up
• Incline Push-up
• Incline Pec Flys
3. Wednesday's Workout (Legs 10 reps per exercise with 4 sets)
• Squat
• Straight-Leg Deadlift
• Hamstring Curl
• Weighted Lunge

4. Thursday's Workout (Shoulders and Arms 10 reps per exercise with 4 sets)

- Incline Biceps Curls
- Triceps Dips
- Lateral Raises
- Shoulder Press

5. Friday's Workout (Power Circuit 10 reps per exercise with 3 sets)

- Clean and Press
- Weighted Knee Raise
- Weighted Step-ups
- Pull up
- Incline Push up
- Triceps Dips

6. Saturday's/Sunday's Workout

- Light cardio such as outdoor/physical activities

Hugh Jackman

Widely known for his long-running roles as the Wolverine in the X-Men film series, as well as various lead roles in movies such as Van Helsing, The Prestige and Les Miserables which got him nominated for Best Actor for the Academy Award. Before he co-starred his role as the Wolverine, he worked together with his trainer David Kingsbury to get his desired shape for the role as the Wolverine. According to his trainer, he was already in a good shape before proceeded to build up his muscle mass and leanness for his role. Due to that, he focused more on direct strength workout with 1-5 rep followed by higher rep schemes.

In order to keep the body percentage low while putting on muscle mass, Hugh Jackman's training mostly consists of both low-intensity and high burst, short training intervals. As a result, he was able to maintain his weight while being shredded with visibly more muscle mass.

He achieved his ideal results from both dieting and performing high-volume of cardio first thing in the morning. So what about the diet? It's actually quite straightforward. On weight training days, he'll consume higher carbs as compared to Off Days and Cardio Days.

In terms of supplement consumption, he took creatine for bulking while for pre and post workout he took BCAAs to preserve lean muscle mass and Universal L- carnitine to help metabolize fatty acids.

Hugh Jackman jumping back into his intensive workout preparing for his upcoming roles in future X-Men sequels

4 Weeks Intensive Training

Hugh's 4 weeks training focuses on progressive overload and keeps striving for personal best. This routine does not encourage sacrificing strength over size because it incorporates both bodybuilding (High Reps, Low/Medium Intensity) and powerlifting styles (Low Reps, High Intensity) of training. This training plan is made up of a 4-week cycle, where you gradually increase the weight each week up to the 3rd week, then drop the heavy weights on week 4 by ~50% and perform high reps instead.

The main lifts include:

- Barbell Bench Press

- Back Squat

- Weighted Pull-Up

- Deadlift

Perform the main lifts first during training days, then proceed with accessories workout of your own choice.

The general outlook of the training schedule is as follows

Week 1
4 sets of 5 reps each
Week 2
4 sets of 4reps each
Week 3
4 sets of 3 reps each
Week 4
4 sets of 10 reps each

Chris Evans

Almost everyone recognizes Chris as Captain America in the movie Avengers and the Human Torch in Fantastic Four. No, it's not like in the movies where you see Chris took some 'wonder drug' to have the Captain America's badass physique. In fact, Chris gained massive amount muscle mass with an intensive workout routine in order to play the role as seen on the silver screen.

His training was mainly focused on resistance training with only minimal cardio which is about 20 minutes a day. Generally, this workout is suitable to those who have been training for over 6 months consecutively and want to shift towards a different workout plan.

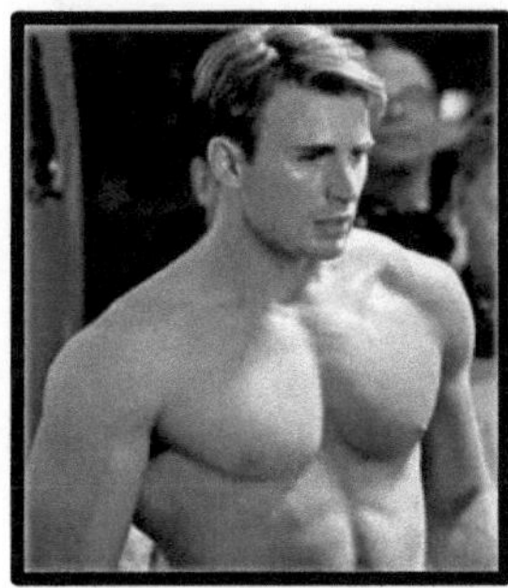

Chris Evans physique during the Captain America: First Avenger film (2011)

Resistance Training Routine

To build up muscle mass, it is recommended to consume whey protein drink about an hour before and after a workout for muscle recovery and growth. The workout routine focuses on 4 sets of each exercise and 8-10 repetitions. Practice 4 sets of each exercise in a row and take a minute rest between each set and before jumping to the next exercise.

Day 1 Shoulders
• Seated Barbell Press
• Lateral Raises
• Dumbbell Press
• Seated Rear Deltoid Raise
• Shrugs
• 10 Minute HIIT Training Session on Treadmill or Bike
Day 2 Chest
• Flat Bench Press

- Incline Chest Press

- Bench Flyes

- Decline Chest Press

- Push-up on Bosu Ball

Day 3 Legs

- Barbell Squats

- Leg Press

- Hack Squats

- Lunges

- Seated Calf Raises

- 10 Minute HIIT Training Session on Treadmill or Bike

Day 4 Arms and Core

- Barbell Bicep Curls

- Skull Crushers

- Incline Seated Bicep Curls

- Cable Hammer Curls

• Dips
• Close-Grip Bench Press
• Ab crunches with legs raised
• 30-second stability ball plank
• Stability ball jackknife
• Oblique crunches on stability ball each side
Day 5 Back
• Pull Ups
• Seated Row
• Lateral Pulldowns
• Stiff Leg Barbell Deadlift
• Bent Over Barbell Row
• 10 Minute HIIT Training Session on Treadmill or Bike
Day 6 and 7 Rest
• Body and energy recovery

Workout Plan For Beginners

For any beginners that would like to start muscle building, the fastest way to see results is to study how the person with the 'ideal' physique you'd die for achieved such result and then leverage such knowledge to achieve a similar result. You really don't have to complicate things nor reinvent the wheels.

The fitness industry has evolved over the years and there are literally countless workout plans out there created by professionals proven to deliver results. All you need to do is to commit to one and follow through, that's it!

Ultimately, there are only 2 Biggest Goals in fitness:

1. Lose Fat
2. Gain Muscles

Again, you only need to decide which are your biggest goal at the moment, choose a workout plan, block out 30, 60 or 90 days… and finally, commit until you achieve your desired body fat percentage or muscle mass.

MUSCLE GAIN SECRET 7

SECRET MUSCLE BUILDING TECHNIQUES FOR VEGANS

The Possibilities Of Building Muscle As A Vegan

As long as you are consuming the right nutrition with high protein, you don't have to be a meat-eater to build muscles. Building up your muscles is 80% from your diet while the remainder 20% comes from your physical exercise and training. To lose fat and build muscle you have to eat correctly. This will be your first and main priority before moving to your physical activities. If you got diet fixed and in check, you are a step closer to building up muscle. That being said building muscle as a vegetarian is a daunting task and a complex one due to the fact you would have a restriction to the certain food that you have access to eat.

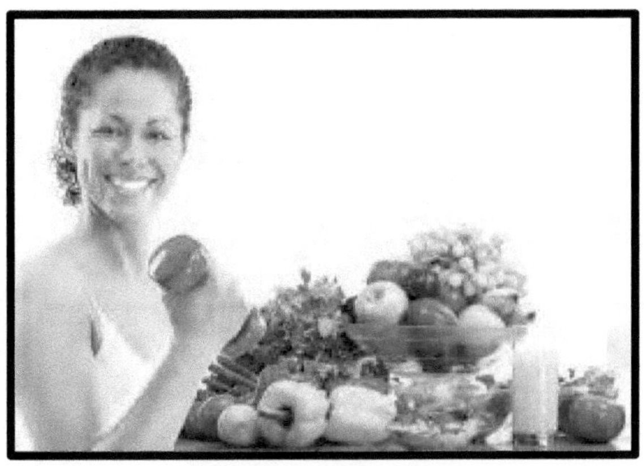

Diet Plan Tip: To build muscle, eat at a surplus and do resistance training

The Essential Nutrients

Determining your vegan diet plan is significant to determine on what you can and should eat and how you can consume it. Just like any ordinary people that have fixed their diet plan, as a vegetarian it is best to track the calories of everything you eat during the entire day. As a vegetarian, your protein requirements will vary from the usual diet plan that ordinary people practice. If you are strength training then you would probably need to take protein supplement with the addition to your personal diet. There are various types of protein based foods that you can consume such as hemp protein, soy, rice protein and gemma protein.

Egg or whey protein are viable options too if you are not a vegan that avoid foods produced by animals or animal products in any way.

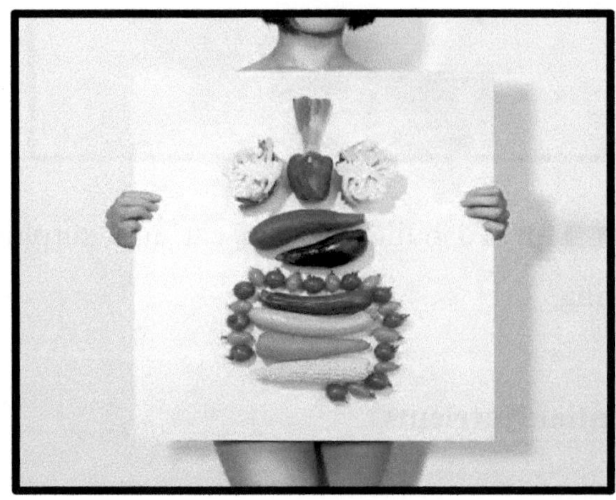

Diet Plan Tip: When it comes to protein consumption, always be conscious of eating various sources of nutrients for a complete distribution of amino acids.

The Significance of Vegetable Protein

There are various significant factors to look into when it comes to the consumption of vegetable protein. Studies showed that the anti-nutritional factors which are commonly found in soy and other vegetable protein have negative effects in human nutrition. These are substances or compound which act to reduce the intake of nutrients, absorption, and utilization and may produce other adverse effects.

Hence, it is highly significant to keep in mind that a higher consumption of vegetable protein is required to gain the same effect of a usual consumption of protein. The best vegetable protein powders you could consider are as followed:

Whey protein: One of the best choices for vegetarians especially for muscle builders. Moreover, it helps with cutting down excess weight and supports the overall of your health. Whey protein can be easily absorbed and digest into your body. Additionally, it is an ideal choice for people who are lactose-intolerant as it tolerable compared to other protein powders. If you're a veganism that is refrained from consuming any dairy products, whey protein is clearly not your choice at is derived from cheese production.

Brown rice protein powder: Is a good option if you can't opt for whey protein as they are gluten and dairy-free. They are packed with high levels of antioxidants and nutrients to support weight loss.

Hemp protein: It contains a complete amino acid profile while it is easy to digest and it helps with pre-workout as it won't cause stomach issues while you are exercising. Moreover, hemp is a safer plant source of protein in general as it is cultivated using the organic agricultural method.

There are various nutrient-dense foods that you can gain protein for your plant-based diet. Vegetables such as avocado, broccoli, spinach, sweet potatoes and boiled peas can be your staple vegan diet. Legumes especially lentils and beans which have been the foundation of various diet plants is a plant that you could consider. They are high in protein and dietary fiber. Moreover, they are mainly feel-good foods for satiety, balancing blood sugar, maintaining weight and energy. Last but not least nuts and seeds can be incorporated into your snack or meal diet plan as they offer high amounts of protein, fiber, vitamins, and minerals.

Planning Out Your Diet!

"Planning out your Diet!" is being self-aware with what you eat and how much you eat daily. The optimized way to do this is to calculate the calories of everything you consume during the course of the entire day with the use of a calorie tracking application or a pen and paper. You can check out https://www.myfitnesspal.com/ to be used a calorie tracker. To easily estimate on how much you should be eating, you need to determine your own Total Daily Energy Expenditure (TDEE). Check out http://www.1percentedge.com/ifcalc/ which is a good tool to adjust your calorie intake to match your personal goal whether that is muscle build-up or fat loss.

Suffice to say if you wish to gain muscle, you basically need to eat over your Total Daily Energy Expenditure (TDEE). If you are losing weight at the same time while building muscles, it is best to remain conservative by staying within 500 calories above or below, respectively. TDEE calculator will only project out the estimated daily caloric needs, hence you need to track your daily calorie intake and compare that to your weight loss/gain to determine a more personalized approach. Adjust your daily intake and reassess for the next few weeks, repeat this step until you are losing weight at the motion determined by your own daily deficit.

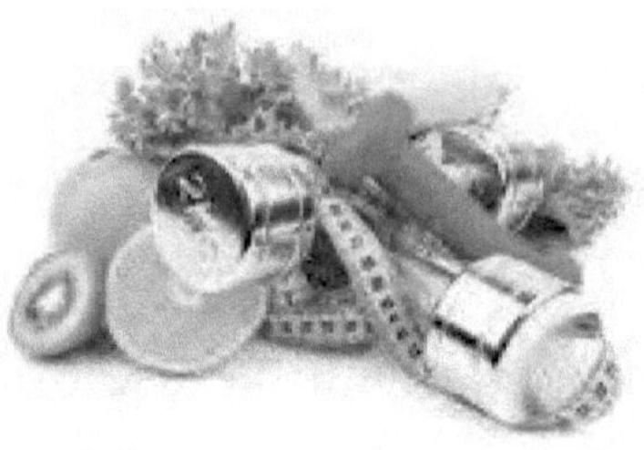

Diet Plan Tip: The best meal plan is always going to be one that you create yourself

Now That The Secret Has Been Revealed

The Great Wall was not built a day. Everything takes time to be better so as your body. As long as you have the determination to carry on, you will definitely taste the sweetness of the fruit by the end of the day. There is no shortcut in building muscle, taking protein powder is just a supplement to help. It is not everything. As I have mentioned in the previous chapter, excessive intake of protein powder will lead to kidney failure and other horrible side effects. You should never risk your health by rushing your body system to achieve what you desire.

Remember, your health is everything. Without healthiness in your life, you are just plain surviving. You are not living it. There is a mere difference between staying a life and living a life. What more can you ask for when you are not able to take a good care of your health? What kind of life do you think you will live without your health? Think about it before you decide to take any shortcuts or any actions.

Printed by Libri Plureos GmbH in Hamburg,
Germany